Hi there!

We're so thrilled you chose us to help you on your chronic illness journey--and what a journey it is.

When we started The Chronic Spoonful Podcast, the need for a planner to track all of our daily needs kept coming up. And we just couldn't find one that did what we wanted.

So, we created one ourselves!

We hope you get out of this what we have. We kept it to a quarter so that it doesn't seem overwhelming to track overthing. When the quarter end, just head back to www.thechronicspoonful.com and pick up your next quarter. Use the code in your reminder email for your discount!!

And don't forget to give us feedback. We know there are other needs out there we can meet. There just aren't enough resources for us, so we want to keep this growing.

Thanks for coming along on this crazy ride with us! We appreciate you, and hope only for the best for you in your journey.

Nicole and Kelli

Hosts

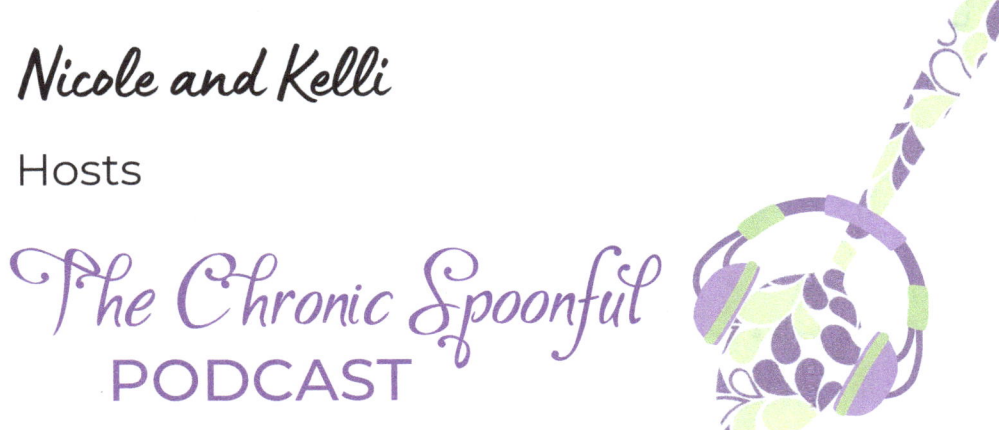

HOW I FELT TODAY

MY SYMPTOMS

- ◯ JOINT PAIN
- ◯ HEADACHE
- ◯ ABDOMINAL PAIN
- ◯ VOMITING
- ◯ LIGHTHEADED
- ◯ FATIGUE
- ◯ BRAIN FOG
- ◯ DIFFICULTY BREATHING

- ◯ NAUSEA
- ◯ INDIGESTION
- ◯ DIZZINESS
- ◯ CONSTIPATED
- ◯ DIARRHEA
- ◯ DISORIENTED
- ◯ RACING HEARTBEAT
- ◯ FACE RASH

OTHER/NOTES: _____

_____

_____

_____

_____

_____

MY WELL-BEING

BODY PAIN	●	●	●	●	●	●	●	●	●
MOOD	😁	☺	😐	☹	😖				
ANXIETY	●	●	●	●	●	●	●	●	●
FATIGUE	●	●	●	●	●	●	●	●	●
BRAIN FOG	●	●	●	●	●	●	●	●	●

NOTES: _____

_____

MY SLEEP

BEDTIME: ____ : ____   ☀ 🌙

WOKE UP: ____ : ____   ☀ 🌙

I WOULD DESCRIBE MY SLEEP AS: _____

_____

_____

WHAT DID I EAT?

Ⓑ · · · · · · · · · · · · · · · · · · ·

Ⓛ · · · · · · · · · · · · · · · · · · ·

Ⓓ · · · · · · · · · · · · · · · · · · ·

Ⓢ

WATER

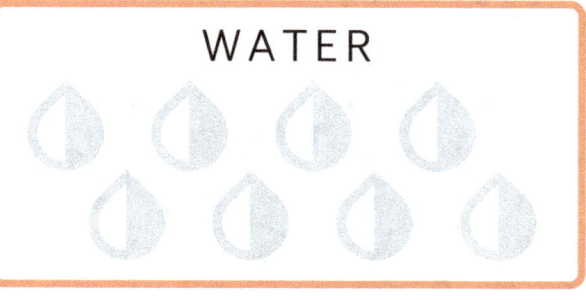

HOW I FELT TODAY

MY SYMPTOMS

- ◯ JOINT PAIN
- ◯ HEADACHE
- ◯ ABDOMINAL PAIN
- ◯ VOMITING
- ◯ LIGHTHEADED
- ◯ FATIGUE
- ◯ BRAIN FOG
- ◯ DIFFICULTY BREATHING

- ◯ NAUSEA
- ◯ INDIGESTION
- ◯ DIZZINESS
- ◯ CONSTIPATED
- ◯ DIARRHEA
- ◯ DISORIENTED
- ◯ RACING HEARTBEAT
- ◯ FACE RASH

OTHER/NOTES: _____

_____

_____

_____

_____

_____

MY WELL-BEING

BODY PAIN	●●●●●●●●●
MOOD	😁 ☺ 😐 🙁 😣
ANXIETY	●●●●●●●●●
FATIGUE	●●●●●●●●●
BRAIN FOG	●●●●●●●●●

NOTES: _____

_____

MY SLEEP

BEDTIME: ___:___ ☀ 🌙

WOKE UP: ___:___ ☀ 🌙

I WOULD DESCRIBE MY SLEEP AS: _____

_____

_____

WHAT DID I EAT?

B ••••••••••••••••••••••••••

L ••••••••••••••••••••••••••

D ••••••••••••••••••••••••••

S

WATER

💧 💧 💧 💧

💧 💧 💧 💧

HOW I FELT TODAY

MY SYMPTOMS

- ◯ JOINT PAIN
- ◯ HEADACHE
- ◯ ABDOMINAL PAIN
- ◯ VOMITING
- ◯ LIGHTHEADED
- ◯ FATIGUE
- ◯ BRAIN FOG
- ◯ DIFFICULTY BREATHING

- ◯ NAUSEA
- ◯ INDIGESTION
- ◯ DIZZINESS
- ◯ CONSTIPATED
- ◯ DIARRHEA
- ◯ DISORIENTED
- ◯ RACING HEARTBEAT
- ◯ FACE RASH

OTHER/NOTES: _____
_____
_____
_____
_____
_____
_____

MY WELL-BEING

BODY PAIN	●●●●●●●●●●
MOOD	😁 🙂 😐 🙁 😆
ANXIETY	●●●●●●●●●●
FATIGUE	●●●●●●●●●●
BRAIN FOG	●●●●●●●●●●

NOTES: _____
_____

MY SLEEP

BEDTIME: ____ : ____ ☀ 🌙

WOKE UP: ____ : ____ ☀ 🌙

I WOULD DESCRIBE MY SLEEP AS: _____
_____
_____

WHAT DID I EAT?

Ⓑ ··
Ⓛ ··
Ⓓ ··
Ⓢ

WATER

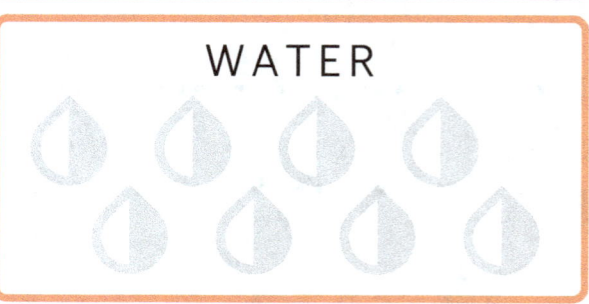

HOW I FELT TODAY

MY SYMPTOMS

- ◯ JOINT PAIN
- ◯ HEADACHE
- ◯ ABDOMINAL PAIN
- ◯ VOMITING
- ◯ LIGHTHEADED
- ◯ FATIGUE
- ◯ BRAIN FOG
- ◯ DIFFICULTY BREATHING

- ◯ NAUSEA
- ◯ INDIGESTION
- ◯ DIZZINESS
- ◯ CONSTIPATED
- ◯ DIARRHEA
- ◯ DISORIENTED
- ◯ RACING HEARTBEAT
- ◯ FACE RASH

OTHER/NOTES: _____

_____

_____

_____

_____

_____

_____

MY WELL-BEING

BODY PAIN	● ● ● ● ● ● ● ●
MOOD	😁 ☺ 😐 ☹ 😣
ANXIETY	● ● ● ● ● ● ● ●
FATIGUE	● ● ● ● ● ● ● ●
BRAIN FOG	● ● ● ● ● ● ● ●

NOTES: _____

_____

MY SLEEP

BEDTIME: _____ : _____ ☀ 🌙

WOKE UP: _____ : _____ ☀ 🌙

I WOULD DESCRIBE MY SLEEP AS: _____

_____

_____

WHAT DID I EAT?

Ⓑ ....

Ⓛ ....

Ⓓ ....

Ⓢ

WATER

💧 💧 💧 💧

💧 💧 💧 💧

HOW I FELT TODAY

MY SYMPTOMS

◯ JOINT PAIN   ◯ NAUSEA

◯ HEADACHE   ◯ INDIGESTION

◯ ABDOMINAL PAIN   ◯ DIZZINESS

◯ VOMITING   ◯ CONSTIPATED

◯ LIGHTHEADED   ◯ DIARRHEA

◯ FATIGUE   ◯ DISORIENTED

◯ BRAIN FOG   ◯ RACING HEARTBEAT

◯ DIFFICULTY BREATHING   ◯ FACE RASH

OTHER/NOTES: _____

_____

_____

_____

_____

_____

_____

MY WELL-BEING

BODY PAIN	● ● ● ● ● ● ● ● ●
MOOD	😁 🙂 😐 🙁 😖
ANXIETY	● ● ● ● ● ● ● ● ●
FATIGUE	● ● ● ● ● ● ● ● ●
BRAIN FOG	● ● ● ● ● ● ● ● ●

NOTES: _____

_____

WHAT DID I EAT?

B ....

L ....

D ....

S

MY SLEEP

BEDTIME: ___:___ ☀ 🌙

WOKE UP: ___:___ ☀ 🌙

I WOULD DESCRIBE MY SLEEP AS: _____

_____

_____

WATER

💧 💧 💧 💧

💧 💧 💧 💧

HOW I FELT TODAY

MY SYMPTOMS

- ◯ JOINT PAIN
- ◯ HEADACHE
- ◯ ABDOMINAL PAIN
- ◯ VOMITING
- ◯ LIGHTHEADED
- ◯ FATIGUE
- ◯ BRAIN FOG
- ◯ DIFFICULTY BREATHING

- ◯ NAUSEA
- ◯ INDIGESTION
- ◯ DIZZINESS
- ◯ CONSTIPATED
- ◯ DIARRHEA
- ◯ DISORIENTED
- ◯ RACING HEARTBEAT
- ◯ FACE RASH

OTHER/NOTES: _____

_____

_____

_____

_____

_____

MY WELL-BEING

BODY PAIN	●●●●●●●●●
MOOD	😁 ☺ 😐 🙁 😣
ANXIETY	●●●●●●●●●
FATIGUE	●●●●●●●●●
BRAIN FOG	●●●●●●●●●

NOTES: _____

_____

MY SLEEP

BEDTIME: ___ : ___ ☀ 🌙

WOKE UP: ___ : ___ ☀ 🌙

I WOULD DESCRIBE MY SLEEP AS: _____

_____

_____

WHAT DID I EAT?

Ⓑ ·····································

Ⓛ ·····································

Ⓓ ·····································

Ⓢ

WATER

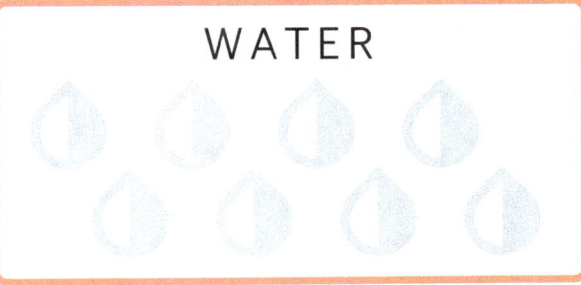

HOW I FELT TODAY

MY SYMPTOMS

- ◯ JOINT PAIN
- ◯ HEADACHE
- ◯ ABDOMINAL PAIN
- ◯ VOMITING
- ◯ LIGHTHEADED
- ◯ FATIGUE
- ◯ BRAIN FOG
- ◯ DIFFICULTY BREATHING

- ◯ NAUSEA
- ◯ INDIGESTION
- ◯ DIZZINESS
- ◯ CONSTIPATED
- ◯ DIARRHEA
- ◯ DISORIENTED
- ◯ RACING HEARTBEAT
- ◯ FACE RASH

OTHER/NOTES:_____

_____

_____

_____

_____

_____

_____

MY WELL-BEING

BODY PAIN	● ● ● ● ● ● ● ● ● ●
MOOD	😁 🙂 😐 🙁 😣
ANXIETY	● ● ● ● ● ● ● ● ● ●
FATIGUE	● ● ● ● ● ● ● ● ● ●
BRAIN FOG	● ● ● ● ● ● ● ● ● ●

NOTES: _____

_____

MY SLEEP

BEDTIME:____:____ ☀ 🌙

WOKE UP:____:____ ☀ 🌙

I WOULD DESCRIBE MY SLEEP AS: _____

_____

_____

WHAT DID I EAT?

Ⓑ •••••••••••••••••••••••••••

Ⓛ •••••••••••••••••••••••••••

Ⓓ •••••••••••••••••••••••••••

Ⓢ

WATER

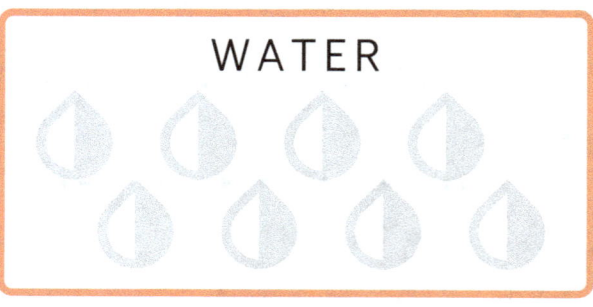

HOW I FELT TODAY

MY SYMPTOMS

- ◯ JOINT PAIN
- ◯ HEADACHE
- ◯ ABDOMINAL PAIN
- ◯ VOMITING
- ◯ LIGHTHEADED
- ◯ FATIGUE
- ◯ BRAIN FOG
- ◯ DIFFICULTY BREATHING
- ◯ NAUSEA
- ◯ INDIGESTION
- ◯ DIZZINESS
- ◯ CONSTIPATED
- ◯ DIARRHEA
- ◯ DISORIENTED
- ◯ RACING HEARTBEAT
- ◯ FACE RASH

OTHER/NOTES: _____

_____

_____

_____

_____

_____

MY WELL-BEING

BODY PAIN	●●●●●●●●●
MOOD	😁 🙂 😐 🙁 😣
ANXIETY	●●●●●●●●●
FATIGUE	●●●●●●●●●
BRAIN FOG	●●●●●●●●●

NOTES: _____

_____

MY SLEEP

BEDTIME: ___ : ___ ☀ 🌙

WOKE UP: ___ : ___ ☀ 🌙

I WOULD DESCRIBE MY SLEEP AS: _____

_____

_____

WHAT DID I EAT?

B ••••••••••••••••••••••••••••

L ••••••••••••••••••••••••••••

D ••••••••••••••••••••••••••••

S

WATER

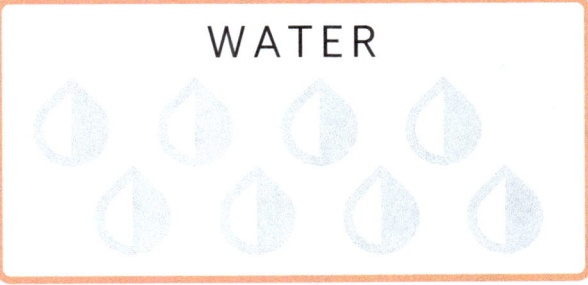

HOW I FELT TODAY

DATE: _____

Ⓜ Ⓣ Ⓦ Ⓣ Ⓕ Ⓢ Ⓢ

WEEK #:   /52

MY SYMPTOMS

◯ JOINT PAIN   ◯ NAUSEA

◯ HEADACHE   ◯ INDIGESTION

◯ ABDOMINAL   ◯ DIZZINESS
   PAIN

◯ VOMITING   ◯ CONSTIPATED

◯ LIGHTHEADED   ◯ DIARRHEA

◯ FATIGUE   ◯ DISORIENTED

◯ BRAIN FOG   ◯ RACING
                        HEARTBEAT

◯ DIFFICULTY   ◯ FACE RASH
   BREATHING

OTHER/NOTES: _____

_____

_____

_____

_____

_____

MY WELL-BEING

BODY PAIN	● ● ● ● ● ● ● ● ●
MOOD	😁 🙂 😐 🙁 😖
ANXIETY	● ● ● ● ● ● ● ● ●
FATIGUE	● ● ● ● ● ● ● ● ●
BRAIN FOG	● ● ● ● ● ● ● ● ●

NOTES: _____

_____

MY SLEEP

BEDTIME: ___:___ ☀ 🌙

WOKE UP: ___:___ ☀ 🌙

I WOULD DESCRIBE MY
SLEEP AS: _____

_____

_____

WHAT DID I EAT?

Ⓑ •

Ⓛ •

Ⓓ •

Ⓢ

WATER

💧 💧 💧 💧

💧 💧 💧 💧

HOW I FELT TODAY

MY SYMPTOMS

- ○ JOINT PAIN
- ○ HEADACHE
- ○ ABDOMINAL PAIN
- ○ VOMITING
- ○ LIGHTHEADED
- ○ FATIGUE
- ○ BRAIN FOG
- ○ DIFFICULTY BREATHING

- ○ NAUSEA
- ○ INDIGESTION
- ○ DIZZINESS
- ○ CONSTIPATED
- ○ DIARRHEA
- ○ DISORIENTED
- ○ RACING HEARTBEAT
- ○ FACE RASH

OTHER/NOTES: _____

_____

_____

_____

_____

_____

MY WELL-BEING

BODY PAIN	● ● ● ● ● ● ● ● ●
MOOD	😁 ☺ 😐 ☹ 😫
ANXIETY	● ● ● ● ● ● ● ● ●
FATIGUE	● ● ● ● ● ● ● ● ●
BRAIN FOG	● ● ● ● ● ● ● ● ●

NOTES: _____

_____

MY SLEEP

BEDTIME: ___:___ ☀ 🌙

WOKE UP: ___:___ ☀ 🌙

I WOULD DESCRIBE MY SLEEP AS: _____

_____

WHAT DID I EAT?

- B ···
- L ···
- D ···
- S

WATER

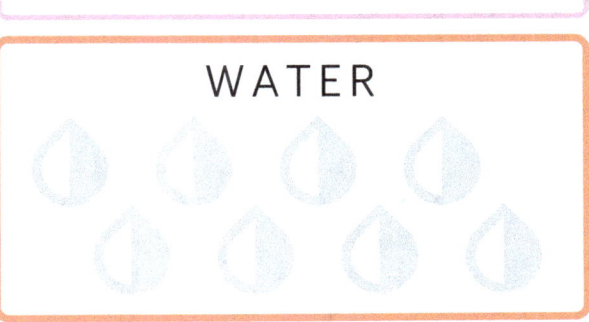

HOW I FELT TODAY

MY SYMPTOMS

- ◯ JOINT PAIN
- ◯ HEADACHE
- ◯ ABDOMINAL PAIN
- ◯ VOMITING
- ◯ LIGHTHEADED
- ◯ FATIGUE
- ◯ BRAIN FOG
- ◯ DIFFICULTY BREATHING

- ◯ NAUSEA
- ◯ INDIGESTION
- ◯ DIZZINESS
- ◯ CONSTIPATED
- ◯ DIARRHEA
- ◯ DISORIENTED
- ◯ RACING HEARTBEAT
- ◯ FACE RASH

OTHER/NOTES: _____

_____

_____

_____

_____

_____

MY WELL-BEING

BODY PAIN	●●●●●●●●●
MOOD	😁 🙂 😐 🙁 😣
ANXIETY	●●●●●●●●●
FATIGUE	●●●●●●●●●
BRAIN FOG	●●●●●●●●●

NOTES: _____

_____

WHAT DID I EAT?

B ....

L ....

D ....

S

MY SLEEP

BEDTIME: ___:___ ☀ 🌙

WOKE UP: ___:___ ☀ 🌙

I WOULD DESCRIBE MY SLEEP AS: _____

_____

_____

WATER

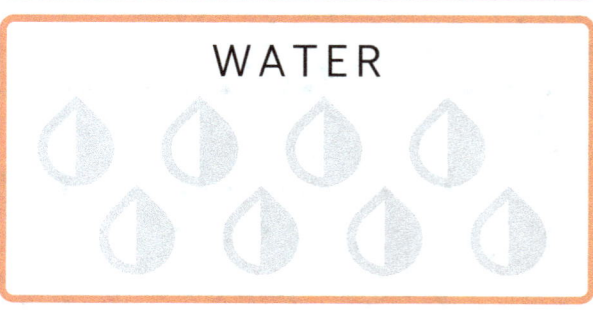

HOW I FELT TODAY

MY SYMPTOMS

- ◯ JOINT PAIN
- ◯ HEADACHE
- ◯ ABDOMINAL PAIN
- ◯ VOMITING
- ◯ LIGHTHEADED
- ◯ FATIGUE
- ◯ BRAIN FOG
- ◯ DIFFICULTY BREATHING

- ◯ NAUSEA
- ◯ INDIGESTION
- ◯ DIZZINESS
- ◯ CONSTIPATED
- ◯ DIARRHEA
- ◯ DISORIENTED
- ◯ RACING HEARTBEAT
- ◯ FACE RASH

OTHER/NOTES:_____

_____

_____

_____

_____

_____

MY WELL-BEING

BODY PAIN	● ● ● ● ● ● ● ●
MOOD	😁 🙂 😐 🙁 😫
ANXIETY	● ● ● ● ● ● ● ●
FATIGUE	● ● ● ● ● ● ● ●
BRAIN FOG	● ● ● ● ● ● ● ●

NOTES: _____

_____

MY SLEEP

BEDTIME: ____:____ ☀ 🌙

WOKE UP: ____:____ ☀ 🌙

I WOULD DESCRIBE MY SLEEP AS: _____

_____

_____

WHAT DID I EAT?

B • • • • • • • • • • • • • • • • • •

L • • • • • • • • • • • • • • • • • •

D • • • • • • • • • • • • • • • • • •

S

WATER

HOW I FELT TODAY

MY SYMPTOMS

- ◯ JOINT PAIN
- ◯ HEADACHE
- ◯ ABDOMINAL PAIN
- ◯ VOMITING
- ◯ LIGHTHEADED
- ◯ FATIGUE
- ◯ BRAIN FOG
- ◯ DIFFICULTY BREATHING

- ◯ NAUSEA
- ◯ INDIGESTION
- ◯ DIZZINESS
- ◯ CONSTIPATED
- ◯ DIARRHEA
- ◯ DISORIENTED
- ◯ RACING HEARTBEAT
- ◯ FACE RASH

OTHER/NOTES:_____

_____

_____

_____

_____

_____

_____

MY WELL-BEING

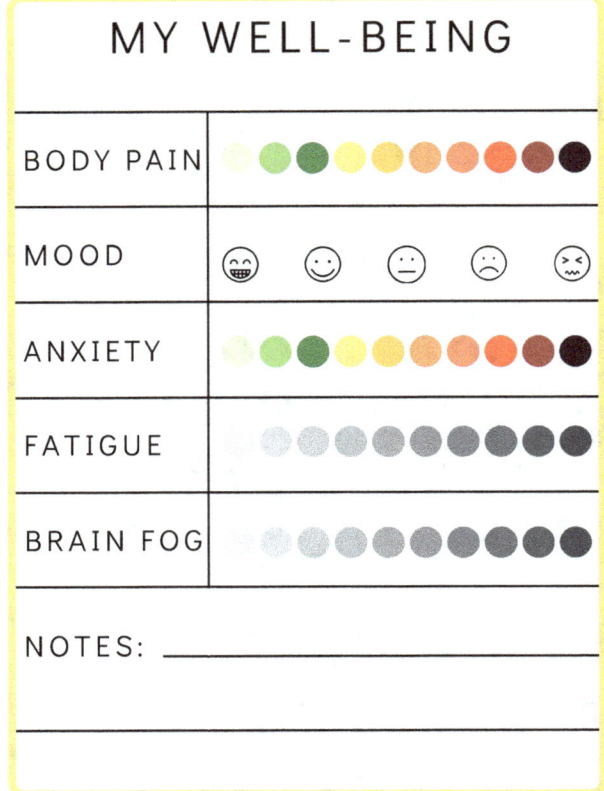

BODY PAIN	
MOOD	
ANXIETY	
FATIGUE	
BRAIN FOG	

NOTES: _____

_____

WHAT DID I EAT?

- Ⓑ •••••••••••••••••••••••••••••
- Ⓛ •••••••••••••••••••••••••••••
- Ⓓ •••••••••••••••••••••••••••••
- Ⓢ

MY SLEEP

BEDTIME: ___ : ___ ☀ 🌙

WOKE UP: ___ : ___ ☀ 🌙

I WOULD DESCRIBE MY SLEEP AS: _____

_____

_____

WATER

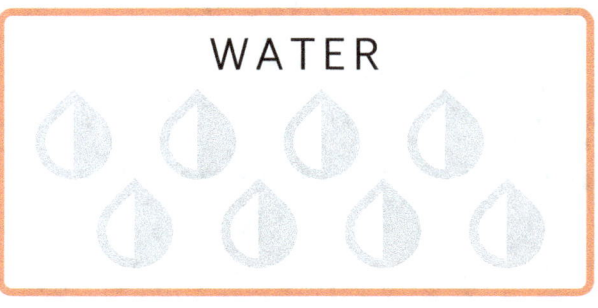

HOW I FELT TODAY

DATE:
_____

M T W T F S S

WEEK #:   /52

MY SYMPTOMS

- ◯ JOINT PAIN
- ◯ HEADACHE
- ◯ ABDOMINAL PAIN
- ◯ VOMITING
- ◯ LIGHTHEADED
- ◯ FATIGUE
- ◯ BRAIN FOG
- ◯ DIFFICULTY BREATHING
- ◯ NAUSEA
- ◯ INDIGESTION
- ◯ DIZZINESS
- ◯ CONSTIPATED
- ◯ DIARRHEA
- ◯ DISORIENTED
- ◯ RACING HEARTBEAT
- ◯ FACE RASH

OTHER/NOTES:_____

_____

_____

_____

_____

_____

MY WELL-BEING

BODY PAIN	●●●●●●●●●
MOOD	😁 ☺ 😐 🙁 😣
ANXIETY	●●●●●●●●●
FATIGUE	●●●●●●●●●
BRAIN FOG	●●●●●●●●●

NOTES: _____

_____

WHAT DID I EAT?

B ··························

L ··························

D ··························

S

MY SLEEP

BEDTIME: ___:___ ☀ 🌙

WOKE UP: ___:___ ☀ 🌙

I WOULD DESCRIBE MY SLEEP AS: _____

_____

WATER

💧 💧 💧 💧

💧 💧 💧 💧

HOW I FELT TODAY

MY SYMPTOMS

◯ JOINT PAIN   ◯ NAUSEA

◯ HEADACHE   ◯ INDIGESTION

◯ ABDOMINAL   ◯ DIZZINESS
   PAIN

◯ VOMITING   ◯ CONSTIPATED

◯ LIGHTHEADED   ◯ DIARRHEA

◯ FATIGUE   ◯ DISORIENTED

◯ BRAIN FOG   ◯ RACING
                         HEARTBEAT

◯ DIFFICULTY   ◯ FACE RASH
   BREATHING

OTHER/NOTES: _____

_____

_____

_____

_____

_____

MY WELL-BEING

BODY PAIN	● ● ● ● ● ● ● ● ●
MOOD	😁 ☺ 😐 ☹ 😖
ANXIETY	● ● ● ● ● ● ● ● ●
FATIGUE	● ● ● ● ● ● ● ● ●
BRAIN FOG	● ● ● ● ● ● ● ● ●

NOTES: _____

_____

MY SLEEP

BEDTIME: ___:___ ☀ 🌙

WOKE UP: ___:___ ☀ 🌙

I WOULD DESCRIBE MY
SLEEP AS: _____

_____

WHAT DID I EAT?

B •

L •

D •

S

WATER

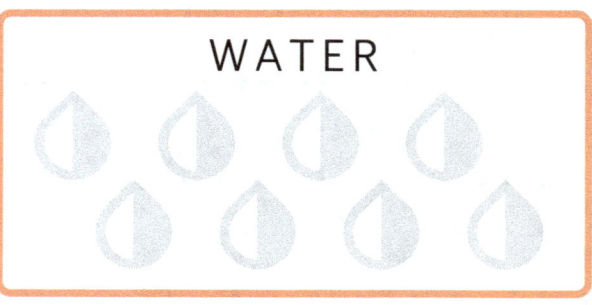

HOW I FELT TODAY

MY SYMPTOMS

- ◯ JOINT PAIN
- ◯ HEADACHE
- ◯ ABDOMINAL PAIN
- ◯ VOMITING
- ◯ LIGHTHEADED
- ◯ FATIGUE
- ◯ BRAIN FOG
- ◯ DIFFICULTY BREATHING

- ◯ NAUSEA
- ◯ INDIGESTION
- ◯ DIZZINESS
- ◯ CONSTIPATED
- ◯ DIARRHEA
- ◯ DISORIENTED
- ◯ RACING HEARTBEAT
- ◯ FACE RASH

OTHER/NOTES: _____

_____

_____

_____

_____

_____

MY WELL-BEING

BODY PAIN	●●●●●●●●●
MOOD	😁 🙂 😐 🙁 😣
ANXIETY	●●●●●●●●●
FATIGUE	●●●●●●●●●
BRAIN FOG	●●●●●●●●●

NOTES: _____

_____

MY SLEEP

BEDTIME: ___:___ ☀ 🌙

WOKE UP: ___:___ ☀ 🌙

I WOULD DESCRIBE MY SLEEP AS: _____

_____

WHAT DID I EAT?

- **B** ....
- **L** ....
- **D** ....
- **S**

WATER

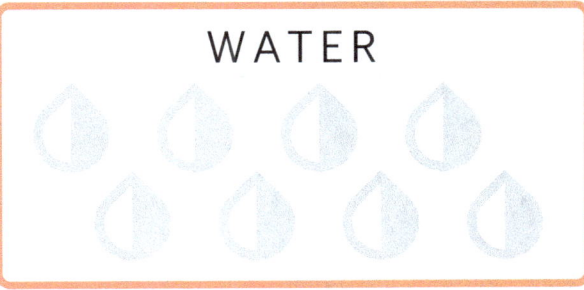

HOW I FELT TODAY

MY SYMPTOMS

- ◯ JOINT PAIN
- ◯ HEADACHE
- ◯ ABDOMINAL PAIN
- ◯ VOMITING
- ◯ LIGHTHEADED
- ◯ FATIGUE
- ◯ BRAIN FOG
- ◯ DIFFICULTY BREATHING

- ◯ NAUSEA
- ◯ INDIGESTION
- ◯ DIZZINESS
- ◯ CONSTIPATED
- ◯ DIARRHEA
- ◯ DISORIENTED
- ◯ RACING HEARTBEAT
- ◯ FACE RASH

OTHER/NOTES: _____

_____

_____

_____

_____

_____

MY WELL-BEING

BODY PAIN	◯◯◯◯◯◯◯◯
MOOD	😁 ☺ 😐 🙁 😫
ANXIETY	◯◯◯◯◯◯◯◯
FATIGUE	◯◯◯◯◯◯◯◯
BRAIN FOG	◯◯◯◯◯◯◯◯

NOTES: _____

_____

MY SLEEP

BEDTIME: ____:____ ☀ 🌙

WOKE UP: ____:____ ☀ 🌙

I WOULD DESCRIBE MY SLEEP AS: _____

_____

WHAT DID I EAT?

B • • • • • • • • • • • • • • • • • • •

L • • • • • • • • • • • • • • • • • • •

D • • • • • • • • • • • • • • • • • • •

S

WATER

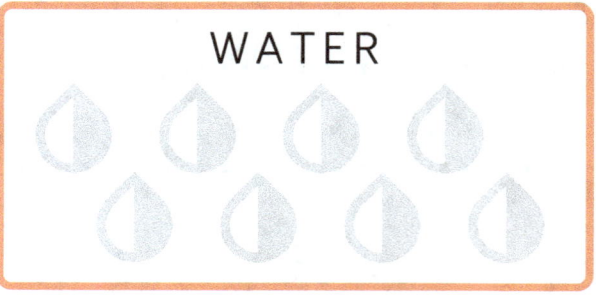

HOW I FELT TODAY

MY SYMPTOMS

- ◯ JOINT PAIN
- ◯ HEADACHE
- ◯ ABDOMINAL PAIN
- ◯ VOMITING
- ◯ LIGHTHEADED
- ◯ FATIGUE
- ◯ BRAIN FOG
- ◯ DIFFICULTY BREATHING

- ◯ NAUSEA
- ◯ INDIGESTION
- ◯ DIZZINESS
- ◯ CONSTIPATED
- ◯ DIARRHEA
- ◯ DISORIENTED
- ◯ RACING HEARTBEAT
- ◯ FACE RASH

OTHER/NOTES: _____

_____

_____

_____

_____

_____

MY WELL-BEING

BODY PAIN	🟢🟢🟡🟡🟠🟠🟠🟤⚫
MOOD	😁 ☺️ 😐 🙁 😣
ANXIETY	🟢🟢🟡🟡🟠🟠🟠🟤⚫
FATIGUE	⚪⚫⚫⚫⚫⚫⚫⚫⚫⚫
BRAIN FOG	⚪⚫⚫⚫⚫⚫⚫⚫⚫⚫

NOTES: _____

_____

MY SLEEP

BEDTIME: ___ : ___ ☀️ 🌙

WOKE UP: ___ : ___ ☀️ 🌙

I WOULD DESCRIBE MY SLEEP AS: _____

_____

_____

WHAT DID I EAT?

Ⓑ ....

Ⓛ ....

Ⓓ ....

Ⓢ

WATER

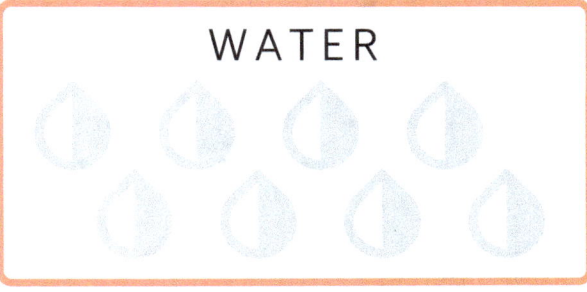

HOW I FELT TODAY

MY SYMPTOMS

- ◯ JOINT PAIN
- ◯ HEADACHE
- ◯ ABDOMINAL PAIN
- ◯ VOMITING
- ◯ LIGHTHEADED
- ◯ FATIGUE
- ◯ BRAIN FOG
- ◯ DIFFICULTY BREATHING

- ◯ NAUSEA
- ◯ INDIGESTION
- ◯ DIZZINESS
- ◯ CONSTIPATED
- ◯ DIARRHEA
- ◯ DISORIENTED
- ◯ RACING HEARTBEAT
- ◯ FACE RASH

OTHER/NOTES: _____

_____

_____

_____

_____

_____

_____

MY WELL-BEING

BODY PAIN	●●●●●●●●●
MOOD	😁 🙂 😐 🙁 😖
ANXIETY	●●●●●●●●●
FATIGUE	●●●●●●●●●
BRAIN FOG	●●●●●●●●●

NOTES: _____

_____

MY SLEEP

BEDTIME: ___:___ ☀ 🌙

WOKE UP: ___:___ ☀ 🌙

I WOULD DESCRIBE MY SLEEP AS: _____

_____

WHAT DID I EAT?

Ⓑ ....

Ⓛ ....

Ⓓ ....

Ⓢ

WATER

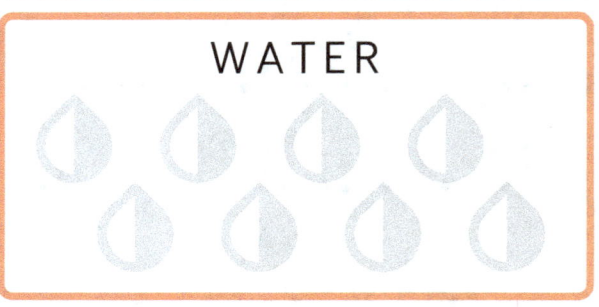

HOW I FELT TODAY

MY SYMPTOMS

- ( ) JOINT PAIN
- ( ) HEADACHE
- ( ) ABDOMINAL PAIN
- ( ) VOMITING
- ( ) LIGHTHEADED
- ( ) FATIGUE
- ( ) BRAIN FOG
- ( ) DIFFICULTY BREATHING
- ( ) NAUSEA
- ( ) INDIGESTION
- ( ) DIZZINESS
- ( ) CONSTIPATED
- ( ) DIARRHEA
- ( ) DISORIENTED
- ( ) RACING HEARTBEAT
- ( ) FACE RASH

OTHER/NOTES: _____

_____

_____

_____

_____

_____

MY WELL-BEING

BODY PAIN	●●●●●●●●●
MOOD	😁 ☺ 😐 ☹ 😖
ANXIETY	●●●●●●●●●
FATIGUE	●●●●●●●●●
BRAIN FOG	●●●●●●●●●

NOTES: _____

_____

MY SLEEP

BEDTIME: ___:___ ☀ 🌙

WOKE UP: ___:___ ☀ 🌙

I WOULD DESCRIBE MY SLEEP AS: _____

_____

_____

WHAT DID I EAT?

B •••••••••••••••••••••••••••

L •••••••••••••••••••••••••••

D •••••••••••••••••••••••••••

S

WATER

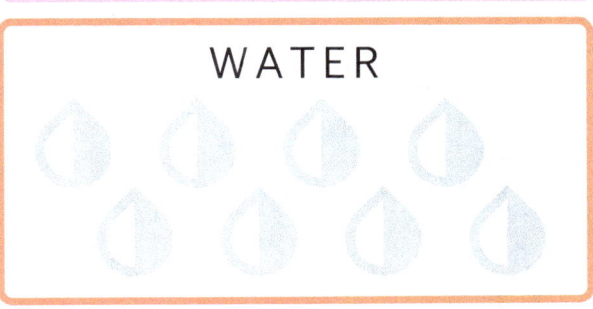

HOW I FELT TODAY

MY SYMPTOMS

- ◯ JOINT PAIN
- ◯ HEADACHE
- ◯ ABDOMINAL PAIN
- ◯ VOMITING
- ◯ LIGHTHEADED
- ◯ FATIGUE
- ◯ BRAIN FOG
- ◯ DIFFICULTY BREATHING

- ◯ NAUSEA
- ◯ INDIGESTION
- ◯ DIZZINESS
- ◯ CONSTIPATED
- ◯ DIARRHEA
- ◯ DISORIENTED
- ◯ RACING HEARTBEAT
- ◯ FACE RASH

OTHER/NOTES: _____

_____

_____

_____

_____

_____

_____

MY WELL-BEING

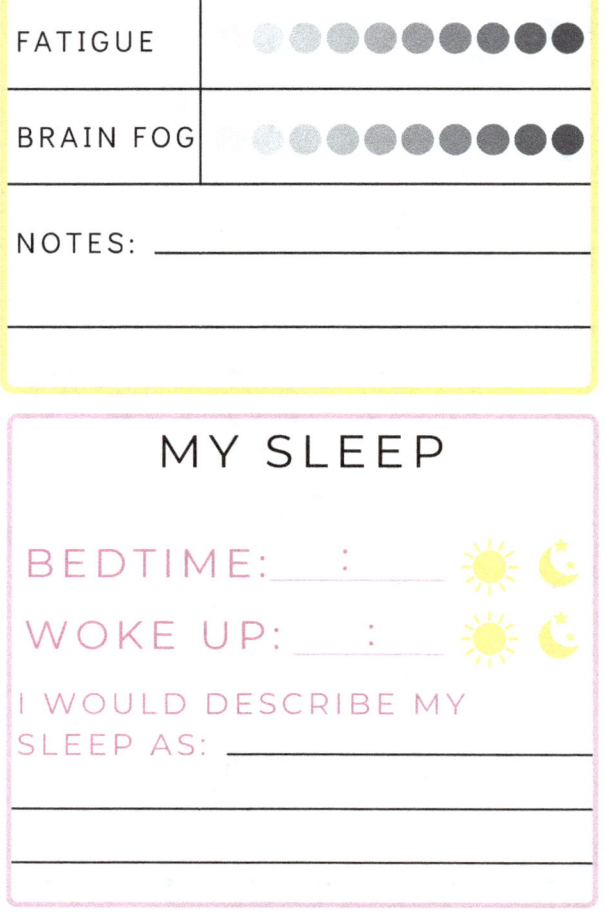

BODY PAIN	
MOOD	
ANXIETY	
FATIGUE	
BRAIN FOG	

NOTES: _____

_____

MY SLEEP

BEDTIME: ____ : ____   ☀ ☾

WOKE UP: ____ : ____   ☀ ☾

I WOULD DESCRIBE MY SLEEP AS: _____

_____

_____

WHAT DID I EAT?

- **B** ....
- **L** ....
- **D** ....
- **S**

WATER

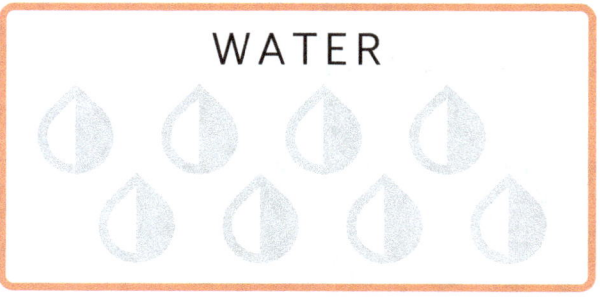

HOW I FELT TODAY

MY SYMPTOMS

◯ JOINT PAIN   ◯ NAUSEA

◯ HEADACHE   ◯ INDIGESTION

◯ ABDOMINAL   ◯ DIZZINESS
  PAIN

◯ VOMITING   ◯ CONSTIPATED

◯ LIGHTHEADED   ◯ DIARRHEA

◯ FATIGUE   ◯ DISORIENTED

◯ BRAIN FOG   ◯ RACING
                     HEARTBEAT

◯ DIFFICULTY   ◯ FACE RASH
  BREATHING

OTHER/NOTES: _____

_____

_____

_____

_____

_____

MY WELL-BEING

BODY PAIN	🟢🟢🟡🟡🟠🟠🟠🟤⚫
MOOD	😁 🙂 😐 🙁 😣
ANXIETY	🟢🟢🟡🟡🟠🟠🟠🟤⚫
FATIGUE	⚪⚫⚫⚫⚫⚫⚫⚫⚫
BRAIN FOG	⚪⚫⚫⚫⚫⚫⚫⚫⚫

NOTES: _____

_____

MY SLEEP

BEDTIME: ____:____ ☀️ 🌙

WOKE UP: ____:____ ☀️ 🌙

I WOULD DESCRIBE MY
SLEEP AS: _____

_____

_____

WHAT DID I EAT?

B •••••••••••••••••••••••••••

L •••••••••••••••••••••••••••

D •••••••••••••••••••••••••••

S

WATER

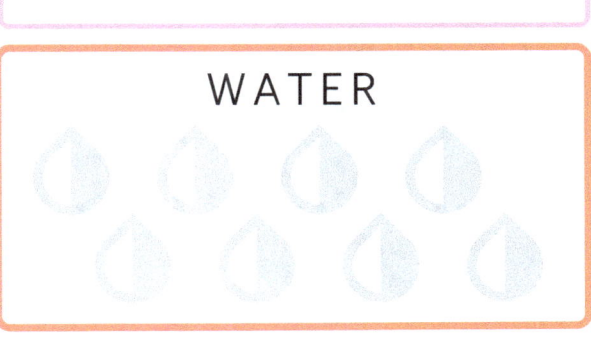

HOW I FELT TODAY

MY SYMPTOMS

- ◯ JOINT PAIN
- ◯ HEADACHE
- ◯ ABDOMINAL PAIN
- ◯ VOMITING
- ◯ LIGHTHEADED
- ◯ FATIGUE
- ◯ BRAIN FOG
- ◯ DIFFICULTY BREATHING

- ◯ NAUSEA
- ◯ INDIGESTION
- ◯ DIZZINESS
- ◯ CONSTIPATED
- ◯ DIARRHEA
- ◯ DISORIENTED
- ◯ RACING HEARTBEAT
- ◯ FACE RASH

OTHER/NOTES: _____

_____

_____

_____

_____

_____

MY WELL-BEING

BODY PAIN	●●●●●●●●●
MOOD	😁 ☺ 😐 ☹ 😣
ANXIETY	●●●●●●●●●
FATIGUE	●●●●●●●●●
BRAIN FOG	●●●●●●●●●

NOTES: _____

WHAT DID I EAT?

B ....

L ....

D ....

S

MY SLEEP

BEDTIME: ___ : ___ ☀ 🌙

WOKE UP: ___ : ___ ☀ 🌙

I WOULD DESCRIBE MY SLEEP AS: _____

_____

_____

WATER

💧 💧 💧 💧

💧 💧 💧 💧

HOW I FELT TODAY

MY SYMPTOMS

- ◯ JOINT PAIN
- ◯ HEADACHE
- ◯ ABDOMINAL PAIN
- ◯ VOMITING
- ◯ LIGHTHEADED
- ◯ FATIGUE
- ◯ BRAIN FOG
- ◯ DIFFICULTY BREATHING

- ◯ NAUSEA
- ◯ INDIGESTION
- ◯ DIZZINESS
- ◯ CONSTIPATED
- ◯ DIARRHEA
- ◯ DISORIENTED
- ◯ RACING HEARTBEAT
- ◯ FACE RASH

OTHER/NOTES: _____

_____

_____

_____

_____

_____

MY WELL-BEING

BODY PAIN	● ● ● ● ● ● ● ●
MOOD	😁 🙂 😐 🙁 😖
ANXIETY	● ● ● ● ● ● ● ●
FATIGUE	● ● ● ● ● ● ● ●
BRAIN FOG	● ● ● ● ● ● ● ●

NOTES: _____

_____

MY SLEEP

BEDTIME: ___ : ___ ☀️ 🌙

WOKE UP: ___ : ___ ☀️ 🌙

I WOULD DESCRIBE MY SLEEP AS: _____

_____

WHAT DID I EAT?

- **B** ·······································
- **L** ·······································
- **D** ·······································
- **S**

WATER

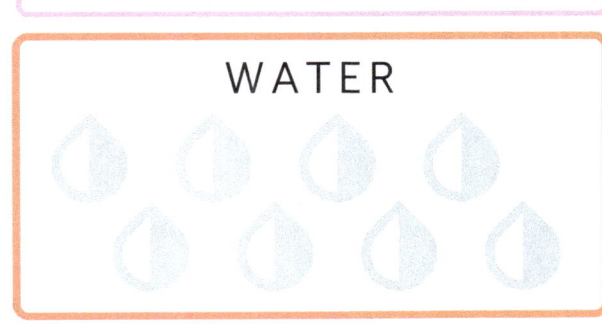

HOW I FELT TODAY

MY SYMPTOMS

- ◯ JOINT PAIN
- ◯ HEADACHE
- ◯ ABDOMINAL PAIN
- ◯ VOMITING
- ◯ LIGHTHEADED
- ◯ FATIGUE
- ◯ BRAIN FOG
- ◯ DIFFICULTY BREATHING

- ◯ NAUSEA
- ◯ INDIGESTION
- ◯ DIZZINESS
- ◯ CONSTIPATED
- ◯ DIARRHEA
- ◯ DISORIENTED
- ◯ RACING HEARTBEAT
- ◯ FACE RASH

OTHER/NOTES: _____

_____

_____

_____

_____

_____

_____

MY WELL-BEING

BODY PAIN	🟢🟢🟢🟡🟡🟠🟠🟤⚫
MOOD	😁 🙂 😐 🙁 😖
ANXIETY	🟢🟢🟢🟡🟡🟠🟠🟤⚫
FATIGUE	⚪⚫⚫⚫⚫⚫⚫⚫⚫
BRAIN FOG	⚪⚫⚫⚫⚫⚫⚫⚫⚫

NOTES: _____

_____

MY SLEEP

BEDTIME: ___ : ___ ☀ 🌙

WOKE UP: ___ : ___ ☀ 🌙

I WOULD DESCRIBE MY SLEEP AS: _____

_____

_____

WHAT DID I EAT?

B •

L •

D •

S

WATER

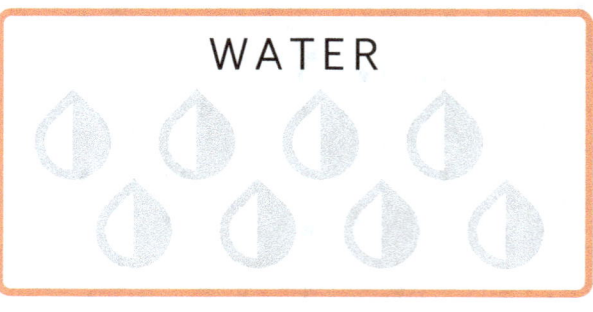

HOW I FELT TODAY

MY SYMPTOMS

- ◯ JOINT PAIN
- ◯ HEADACHE
- ◯ ABDOMINAL PAIN
- ◯ VOMITING
- ◯ LIGHTHEADED
- ◯ FATIGUE
- ◯ BRAIN FOG
- ◯ DIFFICULTY BREATHING

- ◯ NAUSEA
- ◯ INDIGESTION
- ◯ DIZZINESS
- ◯ CONSTIPATED
- ◯ DIARRHEA
- ◯ DISORIENTED
- ◯ RACING HEARTBEAT
- ◯ FACE RASH

OTHER/NOTES: _____

_____

_____

_____

_____

_____

MY WELL-BEING

BODY PAIN	● ● ● ● ● ● ● ● ●
MOOD	😁 ☺ 😐 ☹ 😫
ANXIETY	● ● ● ● ● ● ● ● ●
FATIGUE	● ● ● ● ● ● ● ● ●
BRAIN FOG	● ● ● ● ● ● ● ● ●

NOTES: _____

_____

_____

WHAT DID I EAT?

B •

L •

D •

S

MY SLEEP

BEDTIME: ____ : ____ ☀ 🌙

WOKE UP: ____ : ____ ☀ 🌙

I WOULD DESCRIBE MY SLEEP AS: _____

_____

_____

WATER

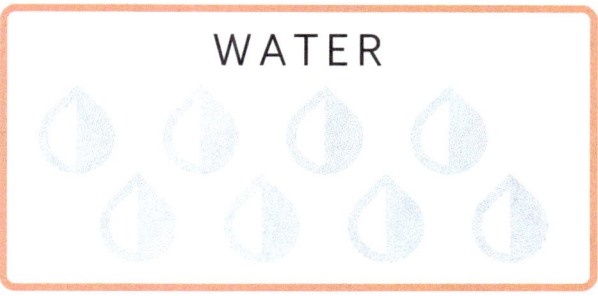

HOW I FELT TODAY

MY SYMPTOMS

- ( ) JOINT PAIN
- ( ) HEADACHE
- ( ) ABDOMINAL PAIN
- ( ) VOMITING
- ( ) LIGHTHEADED
- ( ) FATIGUE
- ( ) BRAIN FOG
- ( ) DIFFICULTY BREATHING

- ( ) NAUSEA
- ( ) INDIGESTION
- ( ) DIZZINESS
- ( ) CONSTIPATED
- ( ) DIARRHEA
- ( ) DISORIENTED
- ( ) RACING HEARTBEAT
- ( ) FACE RASH

OTHER/NOTES: _____

_____

_____

_____

_____

_____

_____

MY WELL-BEING

BODY PAIN	● ● ● ● ● ● ● ● ●
MOOD	😁 🙂 😐 🙁 😣
ANXIETY	● ● ● ● ● ● ● ● ●
FATIGUE	● ● ● ● ● ● ● ● ●
BRAIN FOG	● ● ● ● ● ● ● ● ●

NOTES: _____

_____

WHAT DID I EAT?

B ....

L ....

D ....

S

MY SLEEP

BEDTIME: ____ : ____ ☀ 🌙

WOKE UP: ____ : ____ ☀ 🌙

I WOULD DESCRIBE MY SLEEP AS: _____

_____

_____

WATER

◖ ◖ ◖ ◖

◖ ◖ ◖ ◖

HOW I FELT TODAY

DATE: _____
M T W T F S S

WEEK #: ___ /52

MY SYMPTOMS

- ( ) JOINT PAIN
- ( ) HEADACHE
- ( ) ABDOMINAL PAIN
- ( ) VOMITING
- ( ) LIGHTHEADED
- ( ) FATIGUE
- ( ) BRAIN FOG
- ( ) DIFFICULTY BREATHING

- ( ) NAUSEA
- ( ) INDIGESTION
- ( ) DIZZINESS
- ( ) CONSTIPATED
- ( ) DIARRHEA
- ( ) DISORIENTED
- ( ) RACING HEARTBEAT
- ( ) FACE RASH

OTHER/NOTES: _____

_____

_____

_____

_____

MY WELL-BEING

BODY PAIN	●●●●●●●●●
MOOD	😁 ☺ 😐 🙁 😣
ANXIETY	●●●●●●●●●
FATIGUE	●●●●●●●●●
BRAIN FOG	●●●●●●●●●

NOTES: _____

_____

MY SLEEP

BEDTIME: ___ : ___ ☀ 🌙

WOKE UP: ___ : ___ ☀ 🌙

I WOULD DESCRIBE MY SLEEP AS: _____

_____

WHAT DID I EAT?

- (B) ································
- (L) ································
- (D) ································
- (S)

WATER

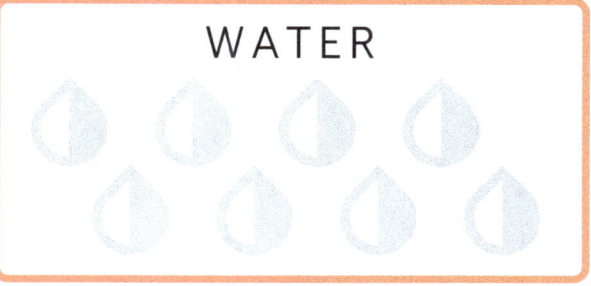

HOW I FELT TODAY

MY SYMPTOMS

- ◯ JOINT PAIN
- ◯ HEADACHE
- ◯ ABDOMINAL PAIN
- ◯ VOMITING
- ◯ LIGHTHEADED
- ◯ FATIGUE
- ◯ BRAIN FOG
- ◯ DIFFICULTY BREATHING

- ◯ NAUSEA
- ◯ INDIGESTION
- ◯ DIZZINESS
- ◯ CONSTIPATED
- ◯ DIARRHEA
- ◯ DISORIENTED
- ◯ RACING HEARTBEAT
- ◯ FACE RASH

OTHER/NOTES: _____

_____

_____

_____

_____

_____

MY WELL-BEING

BODY PAIN	● ● ● ● ● ● ● ● ●
MOOD	😁 ☺ 😐 🙁 😣
ANXIETY	● ● ● ● ● ● ● ● ●
FATIGUE	● ● ● ● ● ● ● ● ●
BRAIN FOG	● ● ● ● ● ● ● ● ●

NOTES: _____

_____

WHAT DID I EAT?

B •••••••••••••••••••••••••

L •••••••••••••••••••••••••

D •••••••••••••••••••••••••

S

MY SLEEP

BEDTIME: ___ : ___ ☀ 🌙

WOKE UP: ___ : ___ ☀ 🌙

I WOULD DESCRIBE MY SLEEP AS: _____

_____

_____

WATER

💧 💧 💧 💧

💧 💧 💧 💧

HOW I FELT TODAY

MY SYMPTOMS

- ◯ JOINT PAIN
- ◯ HEADACHE
- ◯ ABDOMINAL PAIN
- ◯ VOMITING
- ◯ LIGHTHEADED
- ◯ FATIGUE
- ◯ BRAIN FOG
- ◯ DIFFICULTY BREATHING

- ◯ NAUSEA
- ◯ INDIGESTION
- ◯ DIZZINESS
- ◯ CONSTIPATED
- ◯ DIARRHEA
- ◯ DISORIENTED
- ◯ RACING HEARTBEAT
- ◯ FACE RASH

OTHER/NOTES: _____

_____

_____

_____

_____

_____

MY WELL-BEING

BODY PAIN	●●●●●●●●●
MOOD	😁 🙂 😐 🙁 😣
ANXIETY	●●●●●●●●●
FATIGUE	●●●●●●●●●
BRAIN FOG	●●●●●●●●●

NOTES: _____

_____

MY SLEEP

BEDTIME: ___:___ ☀ 🌙

WOKE UP: ___:___ ☀ 🌙

I WOULD DESCRIBE MY SLEEP AS: _____

_____

_____

WHAT DID I EAT?

- B ....
- L ....
- D ....
- S

WATER

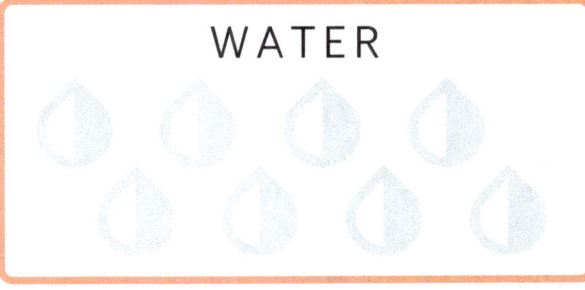

HOW I FELT TODAY

MY SYMPTOMS

◯ JOINT PAIN   ◯ NAUSEA

◯ HEADACHE   ◯ INDIGESTION

◯ ABDOMINAL   ◯ DIZZINESS
   PAIN

◯ VOMITING   ◯ CONSTIPATED

◯ LIGHTHEADED   ◯ DIARRHEA

◯ FATIGUE   ◯ DISORIENTED

◯ BRAIN FOG   ◯ RACING
                         HEARTBEAT

◯ DIFFICULTY   ◯ FACE RASH
   BREATHING

OTHER/NOTES: _____

_____

_____

_____

_____

_____

MY WELL-BEING

BODY PAIN	● ● ● ● ● ● ● ●
MOOD	😁 🙂 😐 🙁 😖
ANXIETY	● ● ● ● ● ● ● ●
FATIGUE	● ● ● ● ● ● ● ●
BRAIN FOG	● ● ● ● ● ● ● ●

NOTES: _____

MY SLEEP

BEDTIME: ____ : ____ ☀️ 🌙

WOKE UP: ____ : ____ ☀️ 🌙

I WOULD DESCRIBE MY
SLEEP AS: _____

_____

WHAT DID I EAT?

Ⓑ ···································

Ⓛ ···································

Ⓓ ···································

Ⓢ

WATER

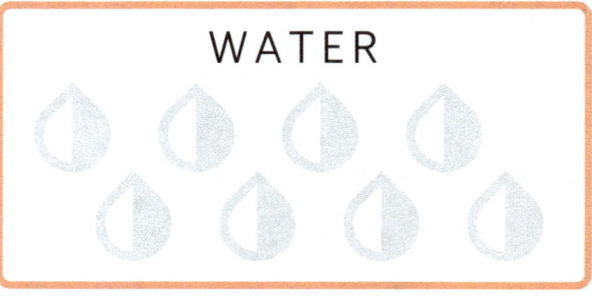

SYMPTOM TRACKER

MONTH: _____   YEAR: _____

SYMPTOM & AREA	1	2	3	4	5	6	7	8	9	10	11	12	13	14	15	16	17	18	19	20	21	22	23	24	25	26	27	28	29	30	31

NOTES:

BLOOD PRESSURE TRACKER

MONTH: YEAR:

SUNDAY	MONDAY	TUESDAY	WEDNESDAY	THURSDAY	FRIDAY	SATURDAY
AM___/___ ♡ ___/___PM ♡	AM___/___ ♡ ___/___PM ♡	AM___/___ ♡ ___/___PM ♡	AM___/___ ♡ ___/___PM ♡	AM___/___ ♡ ___/___PM ♡	AM___/___ ♡ ___/___PM ♡	AM___/___ ♡ ___/___PM ♡
AM___/___ ♡ ___/___PM ♡	AM___/___ ♡ ___/___PM ♡	AM___/___ ♡ ___/___PM ♡	AM___/___ ♡ ___/___PM ♡	AM___/___ ♡ ___/___PM ♡	AM___/___ ♡ ___/___PM ♡	AM___/___ ♡ ___/___PM ♡
AM___/___ ♡ ___/___PM ♡	AM___/___ ♡ ___/___PM ♡	AM___/___ ♡ ___/___PM ♡	AM___/___ ♡ ___/___PM ♡	AM___/___ ♡ ___/___PM ♡	AM___/___ ♡ ___/___PM ♡	AM___/___ ♡ ___/___PM ♡
AM___/___ ♡ ___/___PM ♡	AM___/___ ♡ ___/___PM ♡	AM___/___ ♡ ___/___PM ♡	AM___/___ ♡ ___/___PM ♡	AM___/___ ♡ ___/___PM ♡	AM___/___ ♡ ___/___PM ♡	AM___/___ ♡ ___/___PM ♡
AM___/___ ♡ ___/___PM ♡	AM___/___ ♡ ___/___PM ♡	AM___/___ ♡ ___/___PM ♡	AM___/___ ♡ ___/___PM ♡	AM___/___ ♡ ___/___PM ♡	AM___/___ ♡ ___/___PM ♡	AM___/___ ♡ ___/___PM ♡

BLOOD SUGAR LOG

DATES: _____   **WEEK:** _____

	BREAKFAST			LUNCH			DINNER			SNACK			BEDTIME		
MON															
	BEFORE INSULIN AFTER			BEFORE INSULIN AFTER			BEFORE INSULIN AFTER			BEFORE INSULIN AFTER			BEFORE INSULIN AFTER		
TUE															
	BEFORE INSULIN AFTER			BEFORE INSULIN AFTER			BEFORE INSULIN AFTER			BEFORE INSULIN AFTER			BEFORE INSULIN AFTER		
WED															
	BEFORE INSULIN AFTER			BEFORE INSULIN AFTER			BEFORE INSULIN AFTER			BEFORE INSULIN AFTER			BEFORE INSULIN AFTER		
THU															
	BEFORE INSULIN AFTER			BEFORE INSULIN AFTER			BEFORE INSULIN AFTER			BEFORE INSULIN AFTER			BEFORE INSULIN AFTER		
FRI															
	BEFORE INSULIN AFTER			BEFORE INSULIN AFTER			BEFORE INSULIN AFTER			BEFORE INSULIN AFTER			BEFORE INSULIN AFTER		
SAT															
	BEFORE INSULIN AFTER			BEFORE INSULIN AFTER			BEFORE INSULIN AFTER			BEFORE INSULIN AFTER			BEFORE INSULIN AFTER		
SUN															
	BEFORE INSULIN AFTER			BEFORE INSULIN AFTER			BEFORE INSULIN AFTER			BEFORE INSULIN AFTER			BEFORE INSULIN AFTER		

DATES: _____   **WEEK:** _____

MON															
	BEFORE INSULIN AFTER			BEFORE INSULIN AFTER			BEFORE INSULIN AFTER			BEFORE INSULIN AFTER			BEFORE INSULIN AFTER		
TUE															
	BEFORE INSULIN AFTER			BEFORE INSULIN AFTER			BEFORE INSULIN AFTER			BEFORE INSULIN AFTER			BEFORE INSULIN AFTER		
WED															
	BEFORE INSULIN AFTER			BEFORE INSULIN AFTER			BEFORE INSULIN AFTER			BEFORE INSULIN AFTER			BEFORE INSULIN AFTER		
THU															
	BEFORE INSULIN AFTER			BEFORE INSULIN AFTER			BEFORE INSULIN AFTER			BEFORE INSULIN AFTER			BEFORE INSULIN AFTER		
FRI															
	BEFORE INSULIN AFTER			BEFORE INSULIN AFTER			BEFORE INSULIN AFTER			BEFORE INSULIN AFTER			BEFORE INSULIN AFTER		
SAT															
	BEFORE INSULIN AFTER			BEFORE INSULIN AFTER			BEFORE INSULIN AFTER			BEFORE INSULIN AFTER			BEFORE INSULIN AFTER		
SUN															
	BEFORE INSULIN AFTER			BEFORE INSULIN AFTER			BEFORE INSULIN AFTER			BEFORE INSULIN AFTER			BEFORE INSULIN AFTER		

BLOOD SUGAR LOG

DATES: _____   **WEEK:** _____

	BREAKFAST	LUNCH	DINNER	SNACK	BEDTIME
MON	BEFORE INSULIN AFTER	BEFORE INSULIN AFTER	BEFORE INSULIN AFTER	BEFORE INSULIN AFTER	BEFORE INSULIN AFTER
TUE	BEFORE INSULIN AFTER	BEFORE INSULIN AFTER	BEFORE INSULIN AFTER	BEFORE INSULIN AFTER	BEFORE INSULIN AFTER
WED	BEFORE INSULIN AFTER	BEFORE INSULIN AFTER	BEFORE INSULIN AFTER	BEFORE INSULIN AFTER	BEFORE INSULIN AFTER
THU	BEFORE INSULIN AFTER	BEFORE INSULIN AFTER	BEFORE INSULIN AFTER	BEFORE INSULIN AFTER	BEFORE INSULIN AFTER
FRI	BEFORE INSULIN AFTER	BEFORE INSULIN AFTER	BEFORE INSULIN AFTER	BEFORE INSULIN AFTER	BEFORE INSULIN AFTER
SAT	BEFORE INSULIN AFTER	BEFORE INSULIN AFTER	BEFORE INSULIN AFTER	BEFORE INSULIN AFTER	BEFORE INSULIN AFTER
SUN	BEFORE INSULIN AFTER	BEFORE INSULIN AFTER	BEFORE INSULIN AFTER	BEFORE INSULIN AFTER	BEFORE INSULIN AFTER

DATES: _____   **WEEK:** _____

	BREAKFAST	LUNCH	DINNER	SNACK	BEDTIME
MON	BEFORE INSULIN AFTER	BEFORE INSULIN AFTER	BEFORE INSULIN AFTER	BEFORE INSULIN AFTER	BEFORE INSULIN AFTER
TUE	BEFORE INSULIN AFTER	BEFORE INSULIN AFTER	BEFORE INSULIN AFTER	BEFORE INSULIN AFTER	BEFORE INSULIN AFTER
WED	BEFORE INSULIN AFTER	BEFORE INSULIN AFTER	BEFORE INSULIN AFTER	BEFORE INSULIN AFTER	BEFORE INSULIN AFTER
THU	BEFORE INSULIN AFTER	BEFORE INSULIN AFTER	BEFORE INSULIN AFTER	BEFORE INSULIN AFTER	BEFORE INSULIN AFTER
FRI	BEFORE INSULIN AFTER	BEFORE INSULIN AFTER	BEFORE INSULIN AFTER	BEFORE INSULIN AFTER	BEFORE INSULIN AFTER
SAT	BEFORE INSULIN AFTER	BEFORE INSULIN AFTER	BEFORE INSULIN AFTER	BEFORE INSULIN AFTER	BEFORE INSULIN AFTER
SUN	BEFORE INSULIN AFTER	BEFORE INSULIN AFTER	BEFORE INSULIN AFTER	BEFORE INSULIN AFTER	BEFORE INSULIN AFTER

28 DAY MEAL PLAN

MONTH/DATES: _____

	MON	TUE	WED		FRI	SAT	SUN
WEEK 1	B: L: D:	B: L: D:	B: L: D:	B: L: D:	B: L: D:	B: L: D:	B: L: D:
WEEK 2	B: L: D:	B: L: D:	B: L: D:	B: L: D:	B: L: D:	B: L: D:	B: L: D:
WEEK 3	B: L: D:	B: L: D:	B: L: D:	B: L: D:	B: L: D:	B: L: D:	B: L: D:
WEEK 4	B: L: D:	B: L: D:	B: L: D:	B: L: D:	B: L: D:	B: L: D:	B: L: D:

NEW FOODS:

NOTES

FOOD JOURNAL

DATES: _____

WEEK: _____

FOODS TO LIMIT/CUT

MON
- BREAKFAST
- LUNCH
- DINNER
- SNACKS
- I FELT:

TUE
- BREAKFAST
- LUNCH
- DINNER
- SNACKS
- I FELT:

WED
- BREAKFAST
- LUNCH
- DINNER
- SNACKS
- I FELT:

THU
- BREAKFAST
- LUNCH
- DINNER
- SNACKS
- I FELT:

FRI
- BREAKFAST
- LUNCH
- DINNER
- SNACKS
- I FELT:

SAT
- BREAKFAST
- LUNCH
- DINNER
- SNACKS
- I FELT:

SUN
- BREAKFAST
- LUNCH
- DINNER
- SNACKS
- I FELT:

FOOD JOURNAL

DATES: _____ / _____

WEEK: _____

	MON	TUE	WED	THU	FRI		SUN	FOODS TO LIMIT/CUT
BREAKFAST								
LUNCH								
DINNER								
SNACKS								
I FELT:								

FOOD JOURNAL

WEEK: _____

DATES: _____

	MON	TUE	WED	THU	FRI	SAT	SUN	FOODS TO LIMIT/CUT
BREAKFAST								
LUNCH								
DINNER								
SNACKS								
I FELT:								

FOOD JOURNAL

WEEK:

DATES: _____

	MON	TUE	WED	THU	FRI		SUN	FOODS TO LIMIT/CUT
BREAKFAST								
LUNCH								
DINNER								
SNACKS								
I FELT:								

DAILY WORKOUT LOG

DATE: _____

CARDIO

TYPE	MODE	TIME

WARM UP

COOL DOWN

NON-AEROBIC EXERCISES

EXERCISE	SETS	REPS	WEIGHT

YOGA EXERCISES

POSITION	TIME	DONE
		○
		○
		○
		○
		○
		○
		○
		○

ONE MAY WALK OVER THE HIGHEST
MOUNTAIN ONE STEP AT A TIME
- JOHN WANAMAKER

NOTES

DAILY WORKOUT LOG

DATE: _____

CARDIO

TYPE	MODE	TIME

WARM UP

COOL DOWN

NON-AEROBIC EXERCISES

EXERCISE	SETS	REPS	WEIGHT

YOGA EXERCISES

POSITION	TIME	DONE
		○
		○
		○
		○
		○
		○
		○
		○

ONE MAY WALK OVER THE HIGHEST
MOUNTAIN ONE STEP AT A TIME
- JOHN WANAMAKER

NOTES

DAILY WORKOUT LOG

DATE: _____

CARDIO

TYPE	MODE	TIME

WARM UP

COOL DOWN

NON-AEROBIC EXERCISES

EXERCISE	SETS	REPS	WEIGHT

YOGA EXERCISES

POSITION	TIME	DONE
		○
		○
		○
		○
		○
		○
		○
		○

ONE MAY WALK OVER THE HIGHEST MOUNTAIN ONE STEP AT A TIME
- JOHN WANAMAKER

NOTES

DAILY WORKOUT LOG

DATE: _____

WARM UP

COOL DOWN

CARDIO

TYPE	MODE	TIME

NON-AEROBIC EXERCISES

EXERCISE	SETS	REPS	WEIGHT

YOGA EXERCISES

POSITION	TIME	DONE
		◯
		◯
		◯
		◯
		◯
		◯
		◯
		◯

ONE MAY WALK OVER THE HIGHEST
MOUNTAIN ONE STEP AT A TIME
- JOHN WANAMAKER

NOTES

DAILY WORKOUT LOG

DATE: _____

WARM UP

COOL DOWN

CARDIO

TYPE	MODE	TIME

NON-AEROBIC EXERCISES

EXERCISE	SETS	REPS	WEIGHT

YOGA EXERCISES

POSITION	TIME	DONE
		○
		○
		○
		○
		○
		○
		○
		○

ONE MAY WALK OVER THE HIGHEST
MOUNTAIN ONE STEP AT A TIME
- JOHN WANAMAKER

NOTES

DAILY WORKOUT LOG

DATE: _____

WARM UP

COOL DOWN

CARDIO

TYPE	MODE	TIME

NON-AEROBIC EXERCISES

EXERCISE	SETS	REPS	WEIGHT

YOGA EXERCISES

POSITION	TIME	DONE
		○
		○
		○
		○
		○
		○
		○
		○

ONE MAY WALK OVER THE HIGHEST
MOUNTAIN ONE STEP AT A TIME
- JOHN WANAMAKER

NOTES

DAILY WORKOUT LOG

DATE: _____

WARM UP

COOL DOWN

CARDIO

TYPE	MODE	TIME

NON-AEROBIC EXERCISES

EXERCISE	SETS	REPS	WEIGHT

YOGA EXERCISES

POSITION	TIME	DONE
		○
		○
		○
		○
		○
		○
		○
		○

ONE MAY WALK OVER THE HIGHEST
MOUNTAIN ONE STEP AT A TIME
- JOHN WANAMAKER

NOTES

DAILY WORKOUT LOG

DATE: _____

CARDIO

TYPE	MODE	TIME

WARM UP

COOL DOWN

NON-AEROBIC EXERCISES

EXERCISE	SETS	REPS	WEIGHT

YOGA EXERCISES

POSITION	TIME	DONE
		○
		○
		○
		○
		○
		○
		○
		○

ONE MAY WALK OVER THE HIGHEST
MOUNTAIN ONE STEP AT A TIME
- JOHN WANAMAKER

NOTES

DAILY WORKOUT LOG

DATE: _____

WARM UP

COOL DOWN

CARDIO

TYPE	MODE	TIME

NON-AEROBIC EXERCISES

EXERCISE	SETS	REPS	WEIGHT

YOGA EXERCISES

POSITION	TIME	DONE
		○
		○
		○
		○
		○
		○
		○
		○

ONE MAY WALK OVER THE HIGHEST
MOUNTAIN ONE STEP AT A TIME
- JOHN WANAMAKER

NOTES

DAILY WORKOUT LOG

DATE: _____

CARDIO

TYPE	MODE	TIME

WARM UP

COOL DOWN

NON-AEROBIC EXERCISES

EXERCISE	SETS	REPS	WEIGHT

YOGA EXERCISES

POSITION	TIME	DONE
		○
		○
		○
		○
		○
		○
		○
		○

ONE MAY WALK OVER THE HIGHEST
MOUNTAIN ONE STEP AT A TIME
- JOHN WANAMAKER

NOTES

DAILY WORKOUT LOG

DATE: _____

WARM UP

COOL DOWN

CARDIO

TYPE	MODE	TIME

NON-AEROBIC EXERCISES

EXERCISE	SETS	REPS	WEIGHT

YOGA EXERCISES

POSITION	TIME	DONE
		◯
		◯
		◯
		◯
		◯
		◯
		◯
		◯

ONE MAY WALK OVER THE HIGHEST MOUNTAIN ONE STEP AT A TIME
- JOHN WANAMAKER

NOTES

DAILY WORKOUT LOG

DATE: _____

WARM UP

COOL DOWN

CARDIO

TYPE	MODE	TIME

NON-AEROBIC EXERCISES

EXERCISE	SETS	REPS	WEIGHT

YOGA EXERCISES

POSITION	TIME	DONE
		◯
		◯
		◯
		◯
		◯
		◯
		◯
		◯

ONE MAY WALK OVER THE HIGHEST
MOUNTAIN ONE STEP AT A TIME
- JOHN WANAMAKER

NOTES

DAILY WORKOUT LOG

DATE: _____

WARM UP

COOL DOWN

CARDIO

TYPE	MODE	TIME

NON-AEROBIC EXERCISES

EXERCISE	SETS	REPS	WEIGHT

YOGA EXERCISES

POSITION	TIME	DONE
		○
		○
		○
		○
		○
		○
		○
		○

ONE MAY WALK OVER THE HIGHEST
MOUNTAIN ONE STEP AT A TIME
- JOHN WANAMAKER

NOTES

DAILY WORKOUT LOG

DATE: _____

CARDIO

TYPE	MODE	TIME

WARM UP

COOL DOWN

NON-AEROBIC EXERCISES

EXERCISE	SETS	REPS	WEIGHT

YOGA EXERCISES

POSITION	TIME	DONE
		○
		○
		○
		○
		○
		○
		○
		○

NOTES

ONE MAY WALK OVER THE HIGHEST
MOUNTAIN ONE STEP AT A TIME
- JOHN WANAMAKER

DAILY WORKOUT LOG

DATE: _____

WARM UP

COOL DOWN

CARDIO

TYPE	MODE	TIME

NON-AEROBIC EXERCISES

EXERCISE	SETS	REPS	WEIGHT

YOGA EXERCISES

POSITION	TIME	DONE
		◯
		◯
		◯
		◯
		◯
		◯
		◯
		◯

ONE MAY WALK OVER THE HIGHEST
MOUNTAIN ONE STEP AT A TIME
- JOHN WANAMAKER

NOTES

DAILY WORKOUT LOG

DATE: _____

WARM UP

COOL DOWN

CARDIO

TYPE	MODE	TIME

NON-AEROBIC EXERCISES

EXERCISE	SETS	REPS	WEIGHT

YOGA EXERCISES

POSITION	TIME	DONE
		○
		○
		○
		○
		○
		○
		○
		○

ONE MAY WALK OVER THE HIGHEST
MOUNTAIN ONE STEP AT A TIME
- JOHN WANAMAKER

NOTES

DAILY WORKOUT LOG

DATE: _____

WARM UP

COOL DOWN

CARDIO

TYPE	MODE	TIME

NON-AEROBIC EXERCISES

EXERCISE	SETS	REPS	WEIGHT

YOGA EXERCISES

POSITION	TIME	DONE
		◯
		◯
		◯
		◯
		◯
		◯
		◯
		◯

ONE MAY WALK OVER THE HIGHEST
MOUNTAIN ONE STEP AT A TIME
- JOHN WANAMAKER

NOTES

DAILY WORKOUT LOG

DATE: _____

CARDIO

TYPE	MODE	TIME

WARM UP

COOL DOWN

NON-AEROBIC EXERCISES

EXERCISE	SETS	REPS	WEIGHT

YOGA EXERCISES

POSITION	TIME	DONE
		○
		○
		○
		○
		○
		○
		○
		○

ONE MAY WALK OVER THE HIGHEST MOUNTAIN ONE STEP AT A TIME
- JOHN WANAMAKER

NOTES

DAILY WORKOUT LOG

DATE: _____

WARM UP

COOL DOWN

CARDIO

TYPE	MODE	TIME

NON-AEROBIC EXERCISES

EXERCISE	SETS	REPS	WEIGHT

YOGA EXERCISES

POSITION	TIME	DONE
		○
		○
		○
		○
		○
		○
		○
		○

ONE MAY WALK OVER THE HIGHEST
MOUNTAIN ONE STEP AT A TIME
- JOHN WANAMAKER

NOTES

DAILY WORKOUT LOG

DATE: _____

WARM UP

COOL DOWN

CARDIO

TYPE	MODE	TIME

NON-AEROBIC EXERCISES

EXERCISE	SETS	REPS	WEIGHT

YOGA EXERCISES

POSITION	TIME	DONE
		○
		○
		○
		○
		○
		○
		○
		○

ONE MAY WALK OVER THE HIGHEST
MOUNTAIN ONE STEP AT A TIME
- JOHN WANAMAKER

NOTES

DAILY WORKOUT LOG

DATE: _____

CARDIO

TYPE	MODE	TIME

WARM UP

COOL DOWN

NON-AEROBIC EXERCISES

EXERCISE	SETS	REPS	WEIGHT

YOGA EXERCISES

POSITION	TIME	DONE
		◯
		◯
		◯
		◯
		◯
		◯
		◯
		◯

ONE MAY WALK OVER THE HIGHEST
MOUNTAIN ONE STEP AT A TIME
- JOHN WANAMAKER

NOTES

DAILY WORKOUT LOG

DATE: _____

CARDIO

TYPE	MODE	TIME

WARM UP

COOL DOWN

NON-AEROBIC EXERCISES

EXERCISE	SETS	REPS	WEIGHT

YOGA EXERCISES

POSITION	TIME	DONE
		○
		○
		○
		○
		○
		○
		○
		○

ONE MAY WALK OVER THE HIGHEST
MOUNTAIN ONE STEP AT A TIME
- JOHN WANAMAKER

NOTES

DAILY WORKOUT LOG

DATE: _____

CARDIO

TYPE	MODE	TIME

WARM UP

COOL DOWN

NON-AEROBIC EXERCISES

EXERCISE	SETS	REPS	WEIGHT

YOGA EXERCISES

POSITION	TIME	DONE
		◯
		◯
		◯
		◯
		◯
		◯
		◯
		◯

ONE MAY WALK OVER THE HIGHEST
MOUNTAIN ONE STEP AT A TIME
- JOHN WANAMAKER

NOTES

DAILY WORKOUT LOG

DATE: _____

WARM UP

COOL DOWN

CARDIO

TYPE	MODE	TIME

NON-AEROBIC EXERCISES

EXERCISE	SETS	REPS	WEIGHT

YOGA EXERCISES

POSITION	TIME	DONE
		◯
		◯
		◯
		◯
		◯
		◯
		◯
		◯

ONE MAY WALK OVER THE HIGHEST
MOUNTAIN ONE STEP AT A TIME
- JOHN WANAMAKER

NOTES

DAILY WORKOUT LOG

DATE: _____

WARM UP

COOL DOWN

CARDIO

TYPE	MODE	TIME

NON-AEROBIC EXERCISES

EXERCISE	SETS	REPS	WEIGHT

YOGA EXERCISES

POSITION	TIME	DONE
		○
		○
		○
		○
		○
		○
		○
		○

ONE MAY WALK OVER THE HIGHEST
MOUNTAIN ONE STEP AT A TIME
- JOHN WANAMAKER

NOTES

DAILY WORKOUT LOG

DATE: _____

WARM UP

COOL DOWN

CARDIO

TYPE	MODE	TIME

NON-AEROBIC EXERCISES

EXERCISE	SETS	REPS	WEIGHT

YOGA EXERCISES

POSITION	TIME	DONE
		○
		○
		○
		○
		○
		○
		○
		○

ONE MAY WALK OVER THE HIGHEST MOUNTAIN ONE STEP AT A TIME
- JOHN WANAMAKER

NOTES

DAILY WORKOUT LOG

DATE: _____

CARDIO

TYPE	MODE	TIME

WARM UP

COOL DOWN

NON-AEROBIC EXERCISES

EXERCISE	SETS	REPS	WEIGHT

YOGA EXERCISES

POSITION	TIME	DONE
		○
		○
		○
		○
		○
		○
		○
		○

ONE MAY WALK OVER THE HIGHEST
MOUNTAIN ONE STEP AT A TIME
- JOHN WANAMAKER

NOTES

DAILY WORKOUT LOG

DATE: _____

CARDIO

TYPE	MODE	TIME

WARM UP

COOL DOWN

NON-AEROBIC EXERCISES

EXERCISE	SETS	REPS	WEIGHT

YOGA EXERCISES

POSITION	TIME	DONE
		○
		○
		○
		○
		○
		○
		○
		○

ONE MAY WALK OVER THE HIGHEST MOUNTAIN ONE STEP AT A TIME
- JOHN WANAMAKER

NOTES

DAILY WORKOUT LOG

DATE: _____

CARDIO

TYPE	MODE	TIME

WARM UP

COOL DOWN

NON-AEROBIC EXERCISES

EXERCISE	SETS	REPS	WEIGHT

YOGA EXERCISES

POSITION	TIME	DONE
		◯
		◯
		◯
		◯
		◯
		◯
		◯
		◯

ONE MAY WALK OVER THE HIGHEST
MOUNTAIN ONE STEP AT A TIME
- JOHN WANAMAKER

NOTES

DAILY WORKOUT LOG

DATE: _____

WARM UP

COOL DOWN

CARDIO

TYPE	. MODE	TIME

NON-AEROBIC EXERCISES

EXERCISE	SETS	REPS	WEIGHT

YOGA EXERCISES

POSITION	TIME	DONE
		○
		○
		○
		○
		○
		○
		○
		○

ONE MAY WALK OVER THE HIGHEST MOUNTAIN ONE STEP AT A TIME
- JOHN WANAMAKER

NOTES

DAILY WORKOUT LOG

DATE: _____

WARM UP

COOL DOWN

CARDIO

TYPE	MODE	TIME

NON-AEROBIC EXERCISES

EXERCISE	SETS	REPS	WEIGHT

YOGA EXERCISES

POSITION	TIME	DONE
		◯
		◯
		◯
		◯
		◯
		◯
		◯
		◯

ONE MAY WALK OVER THE HIGHEST
MOUNTAIN ONE STEP AT A TIME
- JOHN WANAMAKER

NOTES

APPOINTMENT CALENDAR

BE GENTLE WITH YOURSELF. YOU'RE DOING THE BEST YOU CAN.

DATE	EVENT

MONTH: ___

M	T	W	T	F	S	S

MONTH: ___

M	T	W	T	F	S	S

MONTH: ___

M	T	W	T	F	S	S

MONTH: ___

M	T	W	T	F	S	S

APPOINTMENT CALENDAR

BE GENTLE WITH YOURSELF. YOU'RE DOING THE BEST YOU CAN.

DATE	EVENT

MONTH: _____

M	T	W	T	F	S	S

MONTH: _____

M	T	W	T	F	S	S

MONTH: _____

M	T	W	T	F	S	S

MONTH: _____

M	T	W	T	F	S	S

APPOINTMENT CALENDAR

BE GENTLE WITH YOURSELF. YOU'RE DOING THE BEST YOU CAN.

DATE	EVENT

MONTH: _____

M	T	W	T	F	S	S

MONTH: _____

M	T	W	T	F	S	S

MONTH: _____

M	T	W	T	F	S	S

MONTH: _____

M	T	W	T	F	S	S

APPOINTMENT CALENDAR

BE GENTLE WITH YOURSELF. YOU'RE DOING THE BEST YOU CAN.

DATE	EVENT

MONTH: _____

M	T	W	T	F	S	S

MONTH: _____

M	T	W	T	F	S	S

MONTH: _____

M	T	W	T	F	S	S

MONTH: _____

M	T	W	T	F	S	S

DOCTOR APPOINTMENTS

DATE	DR.'S NAME	REASON	OUTCOME

DOCTOR APPOINTMENTS

DATE	DR.'S NAME	REASON	OUTCOME

DOCTOR APPOINTMENTS

DATE	DR.'S NAME	REASON	OUTCOME

DOCTOR APPOINTMENTS

DATE	DR.'S NAME	REASON	OUTCOME

DOCTOR Appointments

DATE	DR.'S NAME	REASON	OUTCOME

Doctor Appointments

DATE	DR.'S NAME	REASON	OUTCOME

DOCTOR APPOINTMENTS

DATE	DR.'S NAME	REASON	OUTCOME

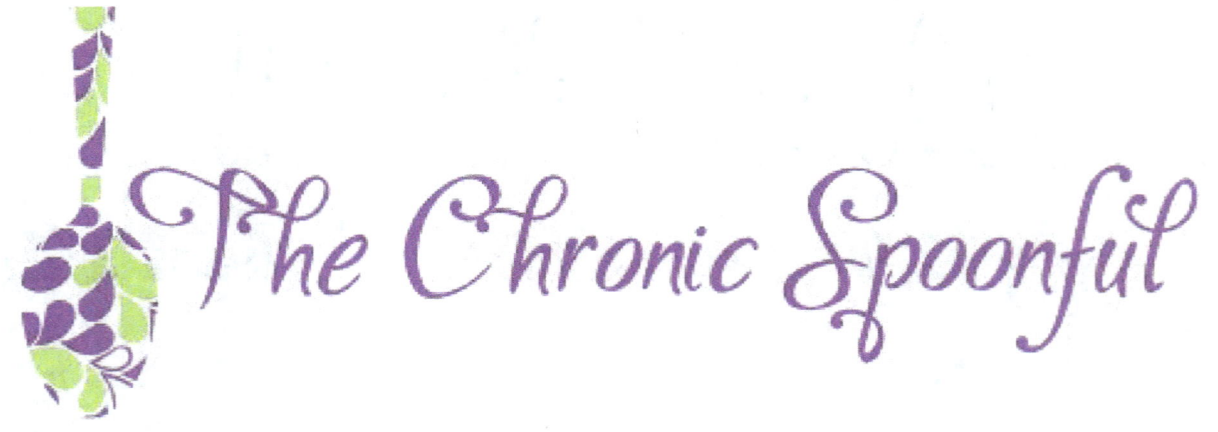

IT'S TIME!!

Head to
www.thechronicspoonful.com
and order your
My Chronic Spoonful Life Planner
for the next quarter!!

www.ingramcontent.com/pod-product-compliance
Lightning Source LLC
Chambersburg PA
CBHW081202280526
45791CB00007B/2164